Life

Life must modulate to circumstances with on emission, to
last.
Has human being, we are in permanent transformation,
evolution, even in revolution in reaction to what we perceived as
reality who itself is irrelevant?

The truth from today, will not be the truth for tomorrow, and vice
versa, think that does not make any sense until now,
can be revealed in the present.

What is valuable and precious for one, would have no value for
somebody else, there is no good or bad, both could be right.
Our mission is simple, to assisted live to what she is doing
best, to maintain living at any cost. Including letting us
swimming in bad water, forcing us facing adversity like a right
of passage to become oneself.

Those resistance are necessary because they resolve to make life
fluid and flexible.
Living is an Art, and QIGONG is a tool, an instrument at
your disposal for creating masterpiece that we have on each
other.

Julie Lagacé

Foreword Jin

The Universe is in perpetual mutation, where thousands of things stir in motion, for the concept of Yin and Yang in their quest for their balance.

always fascinated by oriental philosophy, medicine, and

Martial Art.

There is hundred forms or schools of QIGONG in China, but the 8 of Brocart gave the essence and basic of QIGONG.

The reason for this book is simple, it was the right time for me to say what I must say and do what I must do.

Through this process, I have learned to rely on my own knowledge, intuition, technique, and observations.

Humanity will become more self-relying, self healing, in the future to give more room for celebration and less frustration.

QIGONG really makes me see that as a reality, even if something we stumble in this life.

Gong Fu   continues Works

Canadian Army

My experience in the army was significant. It was like,
an education.

How do we treat each other in the army French Canadian versus?
English?

How do we behave with teamwork, adversity, jealousy?
honor courage and friendship?

Sports Biathlon

I was successful and winning medals in biathlon and
cross-country skiing.

I met nice people, coaches, and athlete from Norway, Russia, and
Canada, who I had the privileged to talk about training, and how
to become a good cross-country skier

Then after a knee injury and because of too much
training and racing,

After six years in the army, it was time for me to try something
different.

For my knee, I have consulted a good Chiropractor who
helped me with my problem, but QIGONG has made the
differences in long terms.
In between, I went back to school and accomplish my degree has
a program leader, tour guide, maintenance guy, massage therapist
and finally discover this marvelous treasure; QIGONG in 2001
Has I been getting older, I put more emphasis on QI GONG,
because of self healing and flexibility.

The advantage of QI GONG!!

-Prevention

-Self-healing process

 -Keep a more stable mind.

-Better flexibility for ligament and muscles

-Release anxiety and stress

-Better understanding of yourself and body function

Doors for energy!!

Our body is scattered with doors of energy, there are situated on the to of your head:
Bahui, at the middle of your hands: Laogong, spinal column Mingmen, vessel belt: hips, Xuehai: knees and under feet:

Yougquan bladder

Those doors are part of the human system, and if you can work with those doors you can be healthier.   QIGONG was great for me. It improves and brings more stability to my knee and more balance in my overall health.
 Do not ask your iPhone to find the answer, those concepts   have been studying for thousands of years, from emperor to martial art, doctors in China and philosopher, just by observing   nature and understanding the link between human, nature, and the Universe.

Therefore, with my student, I try to show them how to open those doors for feeling, balance, and harmony with specific movement.   Not recommended for pregnant woman.

Nature

Nature was always a part of my life as a tour guide and athlete.
Even today, I need to go out regularly to have fresh air to clean up my
mind for preparing my day for planning and put an order in my ideas.

 The mystic always new the necessity for places of high ground,
 like a mountain or a forest. or the pyramids, kind of place to fabric
 new and rebuilt new energy
This process was necessary because, before any great project, you need
to have a reservoir of energy to accomplish certain goal or actions.
 I did experiment this in the Saint James way of Compostela in
Spain in 2011.During long hours of hiking you developed endurance,
 and strength, this trip was rough but educational to me.

Therefore, people who practice QIGONG or Taiichi, are always
near a forest and tree to be in connexion with nature for well
being the worse pollution is the one from people who are not
taking responsibility for their own health.

Protection like a Shield

Your body is essentially made of energy CHI, and your system is a network of meridian or channel. Those channels must be protected.   Imagine an invisible bubble, a (halo) protecting your immune system and the core of your body against negativity, disease, or discomfort of the world.

How I do this!

First asking protection like a form of prayer, in this style: I am asking protection to the silver string, before and after each QIGONG sessions

Visualization and intention

I discover visualization when I was training in biathlon in the army, it helps me to work on my stress before a race
Throughout my own practice in QIGONG and work with my student, the golden sphere, moving the ball and compress the CHI are great movement to build a good immune system

Those who disobey to the law of Universe
Bring, disaster and celestial punishment
But those who respect the law of Universe
Stay healthy from any fatal disease

The classic of oriental medicine
The yellow emperor

Stable mind
 Confucius / Zongzi Confucius said.

First, you must be calm, then your spirit can be stable, when your spirit is stable, then your spirit is in peace. It is only when you are in peace, that you would think clearly and finally win.

What is winning?

Winning is not about control is about revealing what is not Find under the rock why you stopped when you are about to find what was the right thing for you.

We are living in the unstable world, but you do not need to be unstable there is other options, but if you want to stay be unstable this your thing.

One other thing about QIGONG: taking your health is a responsibility, if you want to improve your health with QIGONG, only dedication, time and sweating can improve your health.

Warning be careful about your choice. You can not understand QIGONG intellectually.

Fragile mind (medications like anti-depression) or people with mental health can be affected. Otherwise, you could be caught between conscious- Unconscious and falls perception.

Essence transformation

JING / Fuel, Materials
QI / Energy
SHEN / Spirit

Jing / Fuel, material needed to create and transform your energy throughout your body led with corporeal exercises Vital for the body transformation.

Unlock articulation stretching tendons and muscles facilitated Chi circulations *QI* / energy of the blood, only with a small amount of intention. *Shen / spirit* for guiding and natural movement.

Keep in mind: Jing / Fuel, Qi / Energy- Shen, Spirit, Guidance

Warning:

People with fragile mind (who take medication, anti depressor), or mental health, Be cautious…….

Breathing

6 ways for breathing

1-Natural breathing: maintain your focus on posture and corporeal movement

2-Abdominal respirations: abdomen expand when to inhale and flatten when expiration.

3-Reverse abdominal respiration: the abdomen hollow during inspiration and expand during inspiration.

4-Intentional breathing: intentionally breathing and absorbing fresh air from nature and directed the CHI to specific part of the body

5-Dan Tian breathing: introducing the lower part of the abdomen during breathing

6-Apne Phases: breathing suspended briefly after inspirations. Put your tongue in the palate upper part of your mouth, between your front 2 front teeth and inflate your stomach like a balloon.

In Martial art, you must breath out strongly for a counterattack in a fight, but for QIGONG breathing most be fluidly and silently.

Warm-up

Preparation, prevention is key to be healthy and avoiding injuries, Theories suggests not doing a warmup before an activity.

But I do, it helps in a lot of ways, less injuries more fun and endurance

Personally, I am following The Tui na, and QIGONG for massage therapist in China, they got a selection of reinforcing exercises adaptable for therapist.

Keep your machine in good state and warm up.

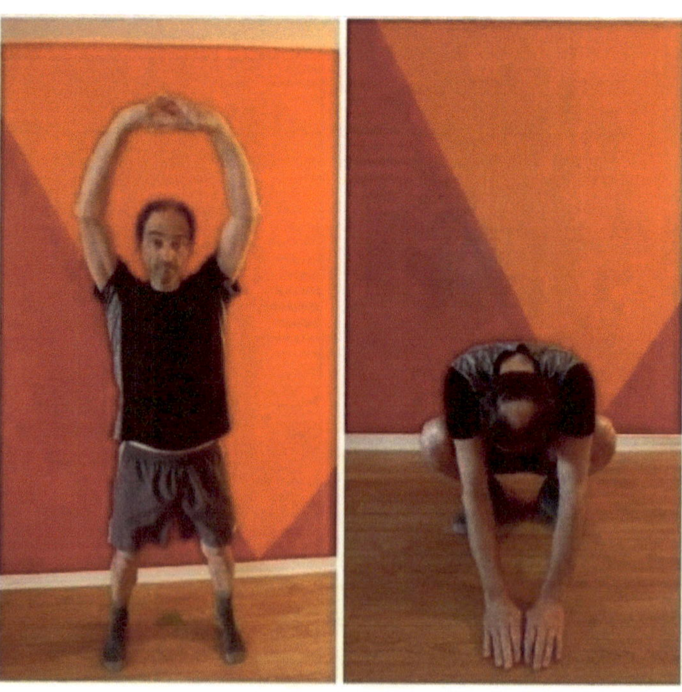

Legs and Posture

Our ancestors were working hard; hunting and farming and they were standing on their two feet, most of the day. Today we spent most of the day sitting at work and not moving too much.

The company and structure in North America are not built for health and prevention, we must do it our self with no time to rest or a meal. Different specialist in another field can see the increase of back problem, diabetes, and obesity.

Working the muscle of your legs are especially important, there is your second heart, legs and hips are stronger than you back, so work your leg regularly.   Stretching and weightlifting can help with your legs otherwise QIGONG can do the work.

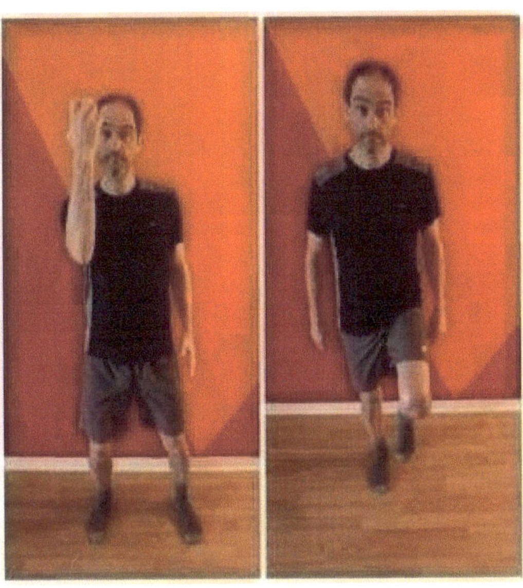

Sowing the Silk

Like the artisan, you need to go back to your work many times with patience and dedication.
Helping the mind to visualize and keep your action in control and relax.

Muscle groups shoulder, arms, neck
Meridians: Triple warmer

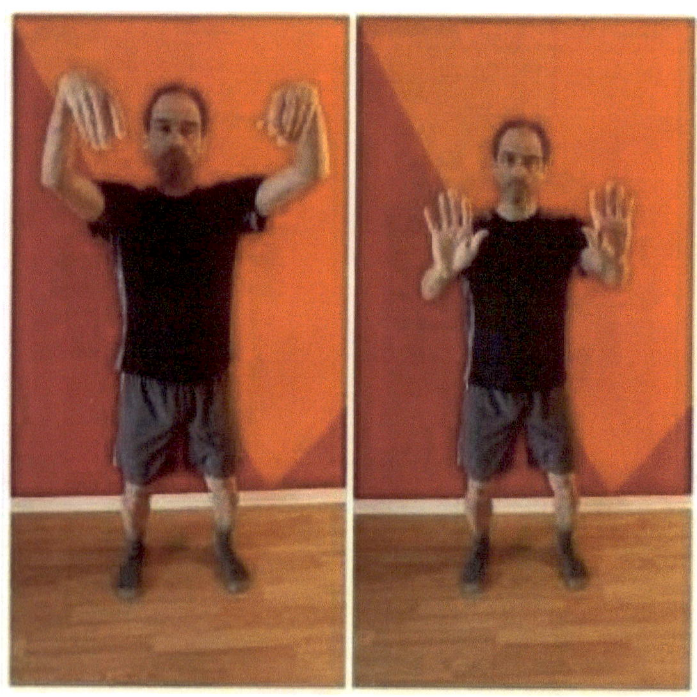

Pushing the Monkey

Like the monkey, you can tease and or be annoying to people around us. I can picture the Monkey like bad emotions, or attitude that emanate from somebody with negative energy, who really want to break your day?

But like the Monkey, you can push this negative energy, away with your hands or with your intentions.

Muscle group: hips, legs, arms
Meridian: K-kidney, B-Bladder

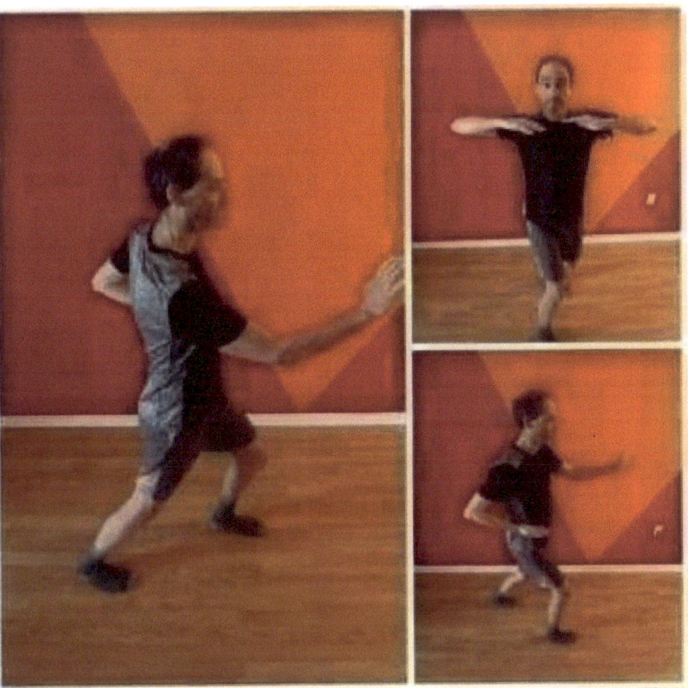

Reaching the Moon
Relax the nervous system, connexion head and back In China, they
call the spine, **the Jade** like the diamond, because the structure of
back and vertebra are precious.
Muscle group: Spine, neck, nervous system

Meridian: Bladder, kidney
Repetitions: both ways right and left 12

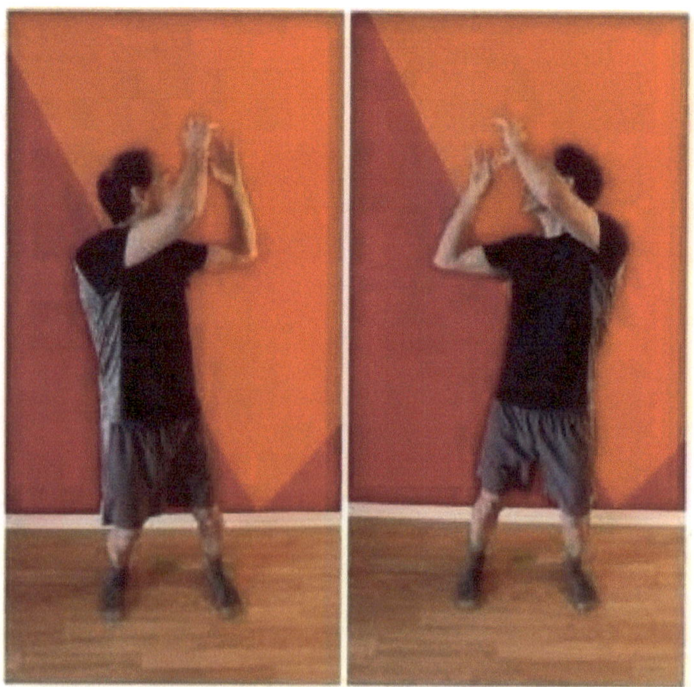

Looking at your rear prevent
5 fatigue and 7 diseases,

like the 5 organs: 5 elements: heart (fire), liver (wood), spleen (earth) kidney (water), lung (metal) a

7 deficiencies: sadness, joy, fear, love, angriness, desire, hatred.

In Chinese medicine, the lack of emotional control can bring disorder, disease, and confusion.

Muscle groups: Legs, hips, arm, neck, nervous system, and head.
Meridian: Liver, Bladder
Repetition 10-12 each side

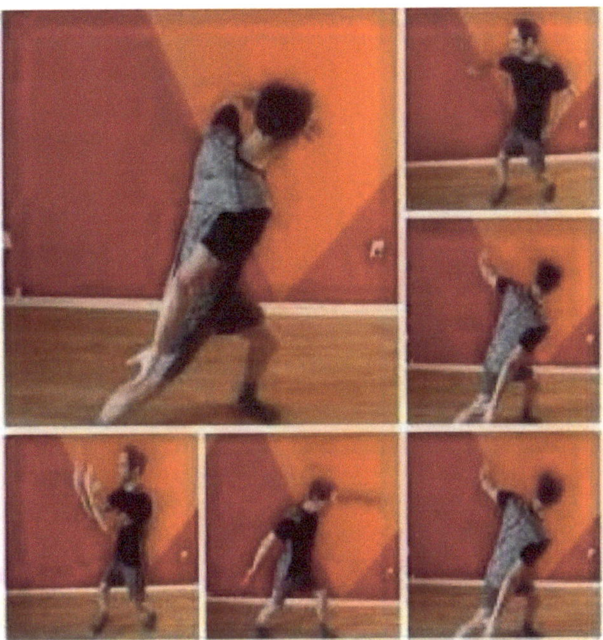

3 pieces of Brocart 19x22 Rise the arms for regularizing the stomach and the spleen.

Help for digestion, and headache, can prevent chronicle disease and good blood circulation

Muscle group: shoulder, biceps
Meridian: Stomach and spleen

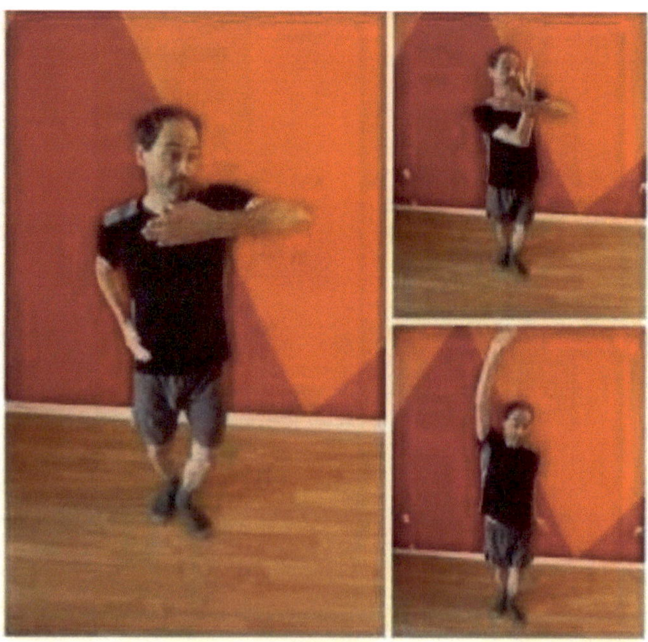

Flexibility

The body and DNA change every second of the day our muscles and tendons change too.
Like our body and muscle, if our mind is rigid, then it will affect your flexibility and your whole body.

There is hundred of exercises and theories about flexibility.

Some say is this not efficient or not good.

But for me it is obvious, I use those who are made for massage therapist in China and Tui na, who give more strength and express oneself with great ease.

Flexibility is something you must work all the time to keep those muscle running, then the whole body is more relaxed.

At his birth, human is soft and flexible
At his death, his stiff and rigid

Alive, plants are full of sap
At Their death, dry and withered
Stiffness and inflexibility have death for a mistress

When life has for discipline, softness, and springiness
**   LAO TSEU**

Cross-country skiing and QI GONG

Unusual, QIGONG can be easily integrated into another form of sports
 Flexibility, visualization, even preparations for races or special
event can be added to specific training.

Therefore, I mixed QIGONG in my preparation for
cross- country skiing training.

QIGONG bring qualities in my techniques thus avoiding injuries.

For that, I am using the Flight of the Crane and another movement to
increase my endurance.

Has a ski patroller, I can see all the time skiers' man and women,
around 75 and 80 years old doing 10 km a day to stay healthy!!

   A good example of longevity

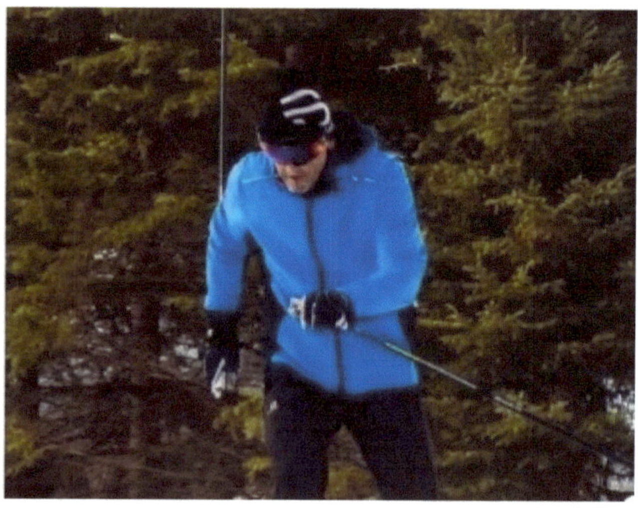

Immune system

Immune system and the moving balls

In ancient China, endurance during a long and hard fight was crucial
for victory or just to stay alive.
Today we do not need to sustain a long fight, but with the moving ball
we can build a stronger immune system.

For that, you must generate enough warm into the body to send the
energy to your channel and internal organ like the bladder and back
and stronger body

Meridian: conceptions vassal, Kidney
Muscle groups: back, arms

**Earth, the sky and I are living in unison: all creation
and I are one identity for which element are inseparable.**

**Chuang Tse
Antique Chinese Philosopher**

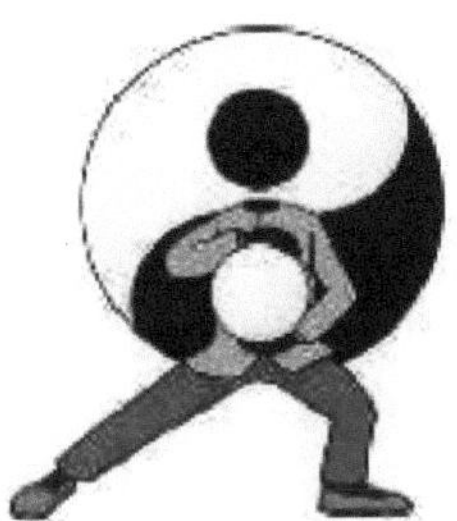

Anxiety stresses, Flight of the crane

Exercise for anxiety, oppression, and heart in the fire. This
simple movement can ease the presser in your shoulder and head.
If you feel oppressed by life, or nothing to seem to go well take 5
minutes!!!
Take the tips of your fingers and touch your shoulders Stress
and anxiety are normal but to feel anxiety and insomnia and
oppression from the world it is not.

Meridian: Bladder, Triple Warmer
Muscle groups: shoulder neck

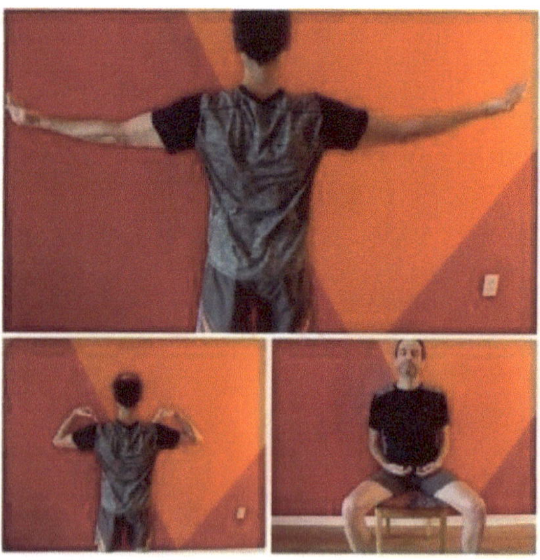

Closing the sessions

I consider the closing of my sessions necessary because interferences can be created around us, sound, emotions, pollution.

At the end of the sessions, I took the Wu Chi stand position.

You are strong but at the same time in peace with yourself

Pictures a river with a strong stream inside you Take a deep breath and let go of the tension.

From time to time, make a follow up in your training.

 Keep track of what you do in a notebook, to see if any variation appears, this way you make changes in your routine and see what work for you.

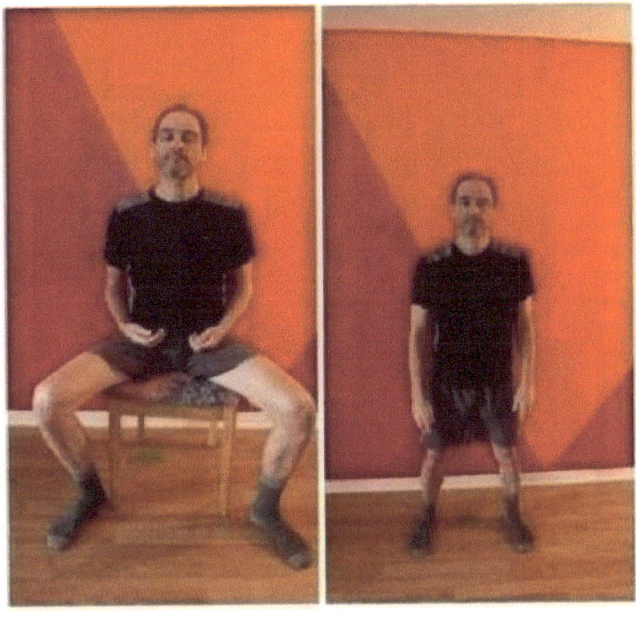

QI GONG and the planet

More and more people are trusting alternative **medicine** all over the planet with: QI GONG, Yoga, meditation, Tachi and acupuncture.

Modern science will have always had a place in civilization, but the population are informed and aware that other form of healing is available with good result in the world, with less medication with more natural medicine.

Imagine, thousands of people doing QIGONG, Yoga, and meditation or what ever, at the same time, and bring more vibrant energy to this planet.

Éric Jouis

References

Voie de Guérison de Dynamisme et de santé

MAITRE LAM KAM CHUEN

QIGONG Dynamique

Maître ANTOINE LY

ZHI NENG QI GONG DE PANG HE MING

Maître ZHOU Jing Hong et Docteur Jean Becchio

QI GONG Le Vol de la Grue

Astrid Schilling et Petra Hintertug

The Author

The author was a professional athlete in biathlon, cross country skiing, and triathlon, was studying biomechanics and concept in long distance training.

The Army has a good impact on his life with experience and discovering himself has a winner, but left with unfinished business, receiving order was not his thing, he was more a freelancer.

After the army he went back to school has a Programme Leader in the tourism, industry, animation, and teacher.

He works with the native community at Manawan and learned their way of life.

He spent time in Silver Star and big white mountain for a job, but never find what he was looking for, but discover QIGONG in 2001, his most profound experience.

Travel to France and Spain the Saint James ways of Compostela. Spirituality, martial arts, Chinese medicine, and nature was always a central part of his personal and professional life.

In 2005 he became a massage and sports therapist,

Essenian and Chinese medicine practitioner, Alzheimer, and challenge person care.

Spirituality is the future of this world, many structures, organizations, groups, and way of thinking will disappear, to gives more room for peace, freedom, and a balance in the Universe.

Table of content